Ultimate Juicing Bible

Complete Guide to Juice Fasting, Detox and Fast weight Loss

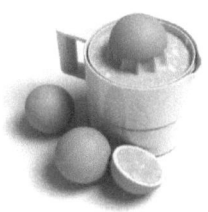

By

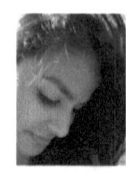

Prianka Mansur

and

Dr. Jacqueline Zaleski Mackenzie

Cover and interior design by: Angela Anderson

Photos were taken from Microsoft clip art and used with permission.

Published by:

CSB Academy

CSB Academy Publishing Co.
P.O. Box 966
Semmes, Alabama 36575

Dedication

I dedicate this book to my mother and others like her who had struggled for years to lose weight with no long-term gain. Women have a much harder time loosing weight than men do. I know that this program works for women because my co-author has faced the same challenges as my mother. This method worked for Jacqueline like none has ever begun to do. May you be as fortunate!

Prianka Mansur

I dedicate this information to those who seek to reduce excess weight. Those people who want to live in a body that offers them endless joy, high self-esteem, and glowing health. This program offers the physical look of health that helps love, respect, income, and public appreciation to flow into you life.

Dr. Jacqueline Zaleski Mackenzie

A personal Thank you from both of us for trying our book, We would love to hear your feedback on Amazon.

To show our appreciation, we have decided to offer everyone that buys our book a free copy of all future update of this book.

Just register your name at:

www.BestJuicingPractice.com

Contents

Preface   - Why we have written this Book

We want to make certain that the public knows the truth about weight loss, health, and fitness; that is why we wrote this book. Juicing is a fast, easy, inexpensive, and natural way to reduce or maintain a good weight/height ratio, overcome numerous diseases, and stay fit for life. We believe that the fear of taking responsibility for your own health and healing in a less conventional manner keeps many people away from seeking natural alternative ways.

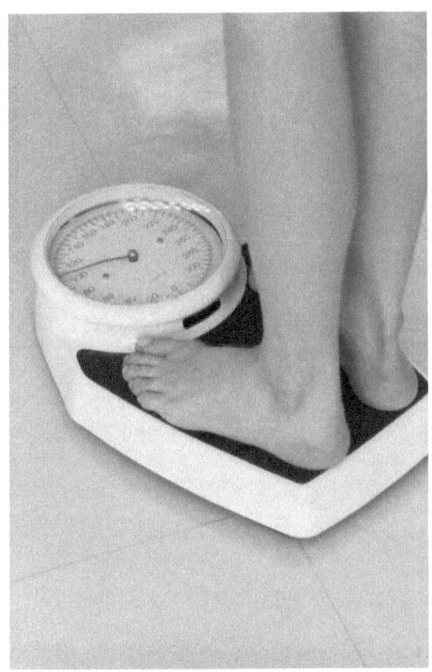

Introduction - Creating a Thin, Healthy, Fit - You

Juicing for weight loss, health, and fitness works. This book will explain why. I will look at scientific research and well as personal testimonials. In each case, you will see that juicing is an easy, inexpensive way to take responsibility for your own weight loss program, cure your body of disease, and be amazed, that in the process, you will look younger and be more energetic.

Alternative healing has high success rates. Nearly $34 billion was spent in 2009 on "complementary and alternative medicine." Although that is only 1.5% of all health care costs (totals about $2.2 trillion), it is 11.2% of out-of-pocket costs.[1] When money is being shelled out, it is clear that a lot of people feel that healing is occurring other than in conventional locations. Instead of spending a great deal of money to add toxins to your body, juicing is inexpensive and removes toxins. Try it and see the results for yourself!

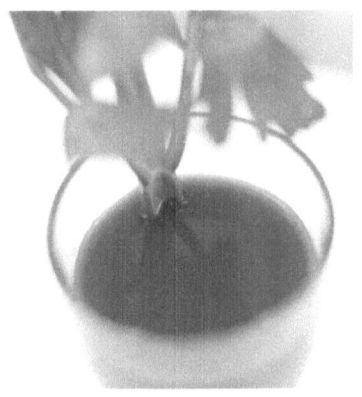

Chapter One - Nothing is Easier

"If you don't do what's best for your body, you're the one who comes up on the short end."

~ Julius Erving

Drinking freshly squeezed juice is a delight for the taste buds. Your digestive system will be relieved that almost no effort is required to turn fresh squeezed juice into energy. Fruit or vegetable juices require almost no effort to digest them. Juices are fat free and yet filling so weight loss is a natural advantage of using juice fasting as a means of encouraging weight loss. Finally, fresh juices, which have not been exposed to heat, offer vitamins, minerals and other natural trace elements to the user. As a result, natural healing occurs. The amount of disease removed from juice fasting seems unreal to most who experience it. No sagging skin or any gaunt appearance results from losing weight by juice fasting.

How Easy Is Juicing?

Juicing or juice fasting is the process of making a blend of several fresh fruits and vegetables to create a fresh drink that is ingested immediately. This process requires a juicer or a specific type of masticating machine that will convert plants including, seeds, and skins into a liquid suitable for drinking. The end fruit juice product can also be diluted with water to create a "fruit water" drink without loosing effectiveness. Typically, vegetable juices are not diluted. The important aspect of this procedure is that the items put into the juicer are fresh and the end result is ingested right away. Live raw plants offer a benefit to the human body that cannot be compared to any other means of seeking weight loss, health benefits or fitness. The rest of this eBook will explain why.

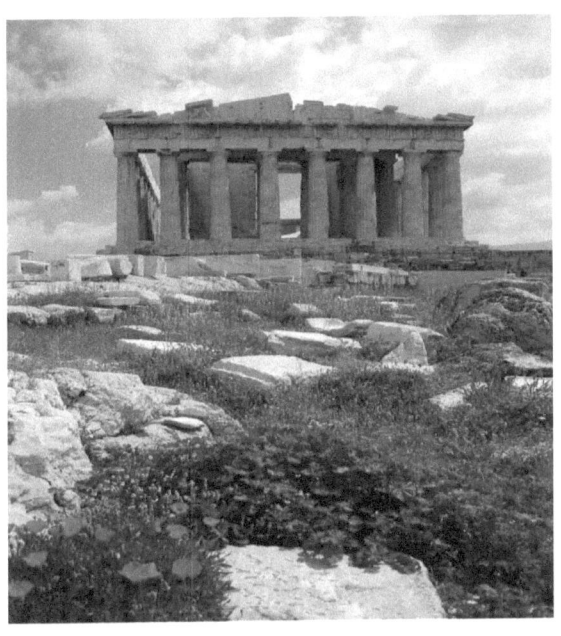

Ancient Physician's Comments Related to Fasting

"Humans live on one-quarter of what they eat;
on the other three-quarters lives their doctor."
~ Egyptian pyramid inscription, 3800 B.C.

"Everyone has a doctor in him or her; we just
have to help it in its work. The natural healing
force within each one of us is the greatest
force in getting well. Our food should be our
medicine. Our medicine should be our food.
But to eat when you are sick, is to feed your
sickness."
~ Hippocrates (Greek) 460 - 370 B.C.E.

Fasting is the greatest remedy, the physician within.
"

~ Paracelsus (Swiss) 1493-1541

Scientific Reports on Juice Fasting

In the 1950's and 1960's, Dr. Lennart Edren lead 325 mile long fasting marches for ten days at 33 miles a day. In each case, the participant's health improved, as did their energy levels. The longest recorded fast was 249 days; the woman was not harmed, but she did lose 74 pounds and her arthritic pain in the process. In 1971, an entire book was devoted to juice fasting, including reporting the recorded scientific research related to fasting.[2]

Currently, awareness of fasting has become a mainstream subject generating increased interest. In March 2012, a report on juice fasting called "Big Gulp" appeared in Time Magazine. The focus was on celebrities using juice fasting as a means to accomplish weight loss, as a means to cleanse the body of toxins, the number of juice fasting cookbooks on the market, and, finally, Starbucks buying juice making firm Evolution Fresh to enable the creation of numerous juice bars around the world. Additionally, the report quoted some skeptical medical doctors who claimed whole body cleansing does not occur during a juice fast.[3]

Is Juice Fasting Going Mainstream?

Now that Starbucks is 40 years old, the newly expanded product line of fresh juice has made a basic difference. Starbucks has changed their logo to reflect this entry into the juice market and the implication is toward healthy food products. The once brown siren with a more prominent mermaid appearance is now bright green, bigger, and the words "Starbucks Coffee" has been dropped. The "Naked" juice will be replaced with the "Evolution Fresh" brand as more health food is introduced into the new Starbuck's stores.[4,5] This is outstanding news for those on a juice fast. Although, juice prepared at home is superior, being able to find deli juice easily is a blessing for those who are working away from home while fasting or who might want to have a meal appointment away from home. This is another example of how easy juice fasting can be.

Fasting has long been a part of religious practices. Studies on fasting have been easy to do because of this isolated group of participants being available. The health results of fasting for religious reasons are not less outstanding than fasting for weight loss, health, or fitness reasons.[6] Attaching more information, it seems that the average person is ignoring doubting medical practitioners and listening to medical doctors who advocate juice fasting.

Consumers, who speak with their wallets, are grabbing juice as meals to lose weight and gain health.

Replacing even one meal (calorie reduction – CR) with fresh juice is beneficial.

> "CR reduces the morbidity of a host of diseases, including (but not limited to), autoimmune diseases, atherosclerosis, cardiomyopathies, cancer, diabetes, renal diseases, neurodegenerative diseases, and respiratory diseases." [7,8]

Intermittent fasting (IF) may be missing only one meal. That activity results in CR has other healthy beauty benefits:

> 'Dietary restriction has been shown to have several health benefits including increased insulin sensitivity, stress resistance, reduced morbidity, and increased life span."[9,10]

Why is Juice Fasting Healthy?

When the digestive system in the human body is not required to work hard to digest food, then the body's resources can be allocated to other activities. The reallocation of resources means that detoxing will likely occur. This process is very good for removing residue from inside the digestive tract. Normally, this detoxing process is noticeable in the form of a thickly coated tongue and bad breath. As the body continues the cleaning process during the fast, the coating is reduced. In most people, when hunger returns the coating is gone and his or her breath is totally without any odor.

Every person is unique. Therefore, the way each body detoxes is different. Some people experience fatigue, body odor, dry skin, pimples, diarrhea, mood swings, confusion, stomachaches, discolored urine, darker than usual bowel movements, insomnia or mucus discharges. For example, one lady reported a great deal of yellow pus-like drainage from a tear duct on her 17th day of a water fast and not a single other symptom until she ended the fast on day 28.

Fasting is a time for reflection as most people find that their clarity of thought is enhanced. Fasting should be a time of careful listening the signals of his or her body and adapting to whatever is going on. His or her body will send clear messages when the fast is complete and the system is clean. Typically day 21 to day 28 is the time frame, but one lady has gone as long as 249 days under careful medical supervision. Trust in natural healing and pay close attention to the parameters of fasting.

How Long is a Juice Fast?

Most people can juice fast for 24 to 36 hours without harmful effects. If you eat dinner of solid foods before 6pm and do not eat solid foods the entire next day until 6pm, a 24-hour fast has been accomplished. During that time, water, herbal tea and fresh raw fruit and vegetable juices are enjoyed. If food is avoided until 6am is reached the second time since stopping eating solid food, a 36-hour fast has been completed. To detoxify normally requires three or more days. Many working people accomplish a three day fast by not eating solid food after lunch on Friday and eating a late very light late lunch the following Monday. A longer fast typically requires the person to consider going to a fasting clinic or to be monitored by a medical professional.

Historically, it is not uncommon for people to fast up to 40 days on water alone and 100 days on juice without any harm. In the words of Dr. Paavo Airola,

"Fasting is one of the safest healing methods known to medical science." [2]

What Counter Indicates Juice Fasting?

People with blood sugar problems are best to avoid water fasting and all fruit juice fasting as regulating blood sugar is a serious issue. Diabetes who are not on medication or insulin may be able to fast for 24-36 hours under medical supervision if the juices are predominately made of vegetables. Check with your medical physician. If a person is a diabetic and also has cancer, the risk of diabetes complications may be overshadowed by the possibility of curing the cancer under medical supervision.

One of the major counter indications to fasting is the taking of medication. Most fasting experts advise that no prescription or over the counter medications should be taken during a fast; that is why being monitored by a medical expert is vital for those typically taking medications. It is also important to avoid topical symptom reducers, toothpaste, mouthwash, deodorant, harsh soaps, face creams, perfumes, and anything else (even vitamins) that might interfere with the body's chemistry or interrupt the natural healing process. Like a newborn baby, your fasting body is busy working to make your circulatory, digestive, endocrine, immune, lymphatic, muscular, nervous, reproductive, respiratory, skeletal, and urinary systems run as perfectly as possible. Harsh chemicals will disrupt that healing, re-balancing process. If in doubt, discuss your normal supplements with an expert.

Any chemicals added to your body may disrupt this process. Consider that even home cleaning products will be passing through your (ungloved) hands or inhaled through your uncovered mouth into your respiratory system. Baking soda is a great cleaning agent for your entire home. A perfectly natural body cleaning option is baking soda; about a teaspoon in a quart to a gallon of water. Use this as a natural means of washing to prevent odors from your mouth, teeth, and entire body. Baking soda and Epson salts is a refreshing bath combination.

How Can Juice Fasting Cure Diseases?

When a person is eating normally, about one-third of the energy from food is fighting the quantity of the additives, chemicals or pollution in the food being eaten. The digestive system, blood, lymph nodes, kidneys, and liver are all working to filter out pollution, chemicals, and other environmental hazards. While busy doing that, the cancer cells are growing unchecked. During a fast, the juice is immediately absorbed; no digestion is required. That time lapse without sorting out waste products and digesting food allows cancer cells to be attacked by the body's own defenses.

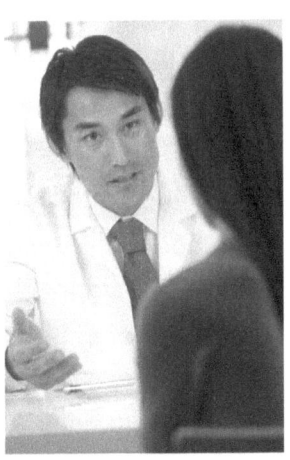

"In my practice I have seen fasting eliminate lupus and arthritis, remove chronic skin conditions such as psoriasis and eczema, heal the digestive tract in patients with ulcerative colitis and Crohn's disease, and quickly eliminate cardiovascular diseases such as high blood pressure and angina. In these cases the recoveries were permanent.

Whether the patient has a cardiac condition, hypertension, autoimmune disease, fibroids, or asthma, he or she must be informed that fasting and natural, plant-based diets are a viable alternative to conventional therapy, and an effective one"

~ ☐Dr. Joel Fuhrman, M.D. author of Fasting And Eating For Health: A Medical Doctor's Program for Conquering Disease

"Fasting is an effective and safe method of detoxifying the body...A technique that wise men have used for centuries to heal the sick. Fast regularly and help the body heal itself and stay well. Give all of your organs a rest. Fasting can help reverse the aging process, and if we use it correctly we will live longer, happier lives.☐Each time you complete a fast, you will feel better. Your body will have a chance to heal and rebuild its immune system by regularly fasting [a major benefit]. You can fight off illness and the degenerative diseases so common in this chemically polluted environment we live in. When you feel a cold or illness coming on or are just depressed-- fast!"

□~ James Balch, M.D. and Phyllis Balch,
C.N.C.

Does Fasting Cure Diseases?

According to a scientific report in February 2012 by Professor Valter Longo of Southern California, "multiple cycles of fasting with chemotherapy cured 20 percent of those (mice) with a highly aggressive form of cancer while 40 percent with a limited spread of the same cancer were cured." He continued to explain: "The cell is, in fact, committing cellar suicide." It appeared that cancerous tumor cells became weaker and more vulnerable during periods of fasting. [11] Dr. Longo's final statement was encouraging:

"A way to beat cancer cells may not be to try to find drugs that kill them specifically, but to confuse them by generating extreme environments, such as fasting, that only normal cells can quickly respond to." [11]

There are stories on the Internet of people who say that fasting cured their cancer.[12] Since cancer is not one, but many aspects of the same run-away growth, it might be helpful to read a few of them. Perhaps purchase Beata Bishop's book, A Time To Heal.

Take a long look at the Gerson Therapy and why it is the means to healing that Ms. Bishop chose to follow.[13] In 1946, Dr. Max Gerson presented his program to a US Congressional Committee, but he lost by four votes to surgery, radiation, and chemotherapy lobbies.[14] Consider the facts, then answer the question "Does fasting cure diseases?" based on what you think about what formerly dying people and scientists are saying.

"For the future of coming generations, I think it is high time that we change our agriculture and our food preservation methods. Otherwise, we will have to increase our institutions for mental patients yearly, and we will see the hospitals overcrowded with degenerative diseases even more rapidly and in greater numbers than the hospitals themselves can be enlarged. I fear that it will not be possible, at least in the near future, to repair all the damage that modern agriculture and civilization have brought to our lives."

~ Dr. Max Gerson

Many scientists have written about the benefits of fasting for physical diseases. However, a few, like Dr. Gerson, had amazing results with drastic mental illness improvements after fasting.[14] Speculation has been that food or food processing allergies have caused or enabled physical or mental illness to continue and that during fasting those irritants have been removed. Dr. Don Colbert strongly advocates juice fasting for that reason.[15] Other scientists feel that during a fast, overall healing includes mental illness. Regardless, healing is the result of fasting. [14]

Chapter Two - Visualize Yourself Thin

"Any experience can be transformed into something of value. Everything depends on the way you look at things. You cannot have the success without the failures."

~ Vash Young

The only way to lose weight is by making the decision to follow a plan of improvement and staying with it long enough to see results. Then making the decision to stay with that plan for life. Think about a ladder or a step machine. Every time you move up you get higher, stepping down is easier, but you lose a physical and a visual advantage in the process of stepping down.

Each time you lose weight, you gain physical health, visual joy in the form of self-esteem, and mental calmness. There is a sense of processing self-control, of having power over how you feel and the way you look. There is no "diet" that can give you that, only a change in how you live. By making juice fasting a way of life, your life will become the life you always dreamed of having.

"It comes down to a simple question: what do you want out of life, and what are you willing to do to get it?"

~ unknown

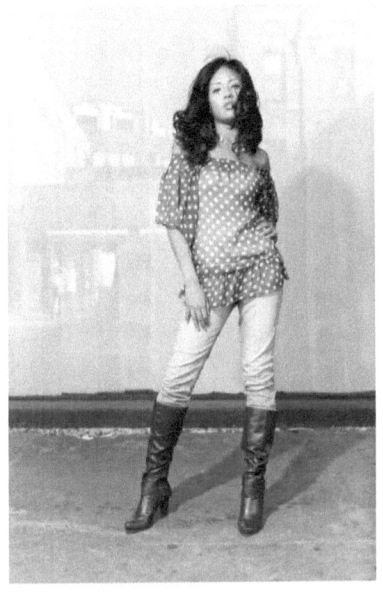

Is Fasting A Safe Weight Loss Option?

Two authors who have used fasting for many years as a means to obtain an ideal weight to height balance and to be disease free are writing this book. Sharing our life experiences is a joy because we wish to be mentors for those who want to be free from the bonds of excess physical bulk and the dangers it can cause to the human carrying it around. Therefore, we offer here comments by medical professionals who agree with our standpoint:

"Fasting is a valid experience. It can benefit any otherwise healthy person whose calories now have the upper hand in his/her life."

~ The New England Journal of Medicine

"Dr. Norman Walker (1886 -1995) was "the" pioneer in the field of vegetable juicing for nutritional health. His book 'Natural Weight Control (1981)' advocated juice fasting for weight management."

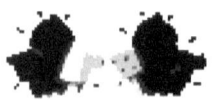 **Easy, Safe, and Healthy – Let's Go!**

There is nothing complicated about juice fasting once you have a real juicer. Trying to make juice by hand or with a conventional blender is a waste of food, electricity, and will power. You will become very frustrated and not end up with a glass of juice. Instead, for about the cost of one month at a local gym or a day at a fancy health spa, you will own a worthwhile juicer. This one piece of equipment is the primary investment in your health.

In the same way that football, horse training, or sailing "experts" have strong opinions, so do those who are avid juicers or raw food advocates have very strong considerations related to juicing. Some juicers prefer pressed juice; others praise low speed juicers (as to not heat the food too much). Many like the classic masticating juicers, and others look at more modern whole food squeezing/masticating/blending; still others add fresh spring water. As time passes, and you evaluate your own results related to weight loss, overall health, and fitness, you too are likely to prefer one method of juicing over another. Everyone needs to pay attention to his or her own body and adapt accordingly. Strong opinions imply that one size fits all, and we all know that is rarely the case.

With most juicers, the fiber is separated during the juicing process. That fiber is good for you. Fiber is a perfect basis for hot or cold soup, to make crackers in a dehydrator or as animal feed. For example, ducks, chickens, and rabbits leap toward a dish of fruit or vegetable fiber. The pulp can also be added to salads, salsas, veggie burgers/meatballs/meatloaf, baked goods or pancake recipes (to make the final baked item more moist), dips, sauces, frozen ice pops for children or ice cubs for adult drinks, baked casseroles or lasagna, and added to a smoothie like raw oats. Think of pulp like adding a few nuts, flax seeds, or nuts to cereal or baked good recipes.

The vital aspects of juicing are (1) in most cases, juice the whole item with skin and seeds (the exception is citrus peel),(2) add more fresh greens as your body will tolerate them, and (3) do not overdo fruit as all that natural sugar can cause blood sugar imbalances.

Consider the following types of juicers:

- A **Manual Juicer** will press or crush one half of a lime, lemon or grapefruit and leave the pulp behind.[17]

- A **Centrifugal Juicer** spins the fruit or vegetable against a blade; they often overheat the juice.[17]

- A **Masticating Juicer** "chews" the fresh produce much like human teeth; typically this is considered the classic.[17]

- A newer **Single Auger Juicer** prevents heating the produce to better preserve the nutritional quality of the product as the juice is both squeezed and pressed.[17]

- A newer **Triturating or Twin Gear Juicer** uses intermeshing twin gears to squeeze and press the produce for both higher yield and better nutritional value.[17]

You do get what you pay for in a juicer. There are many inexpensive home models on the market. Most of them will overheat the motor and your food if you are making enough juice for a fasting diet. However, like exercise equipment, if owning a quality piece of equipment that does not overheat itself or your food is important, then an outstanding option is to buy an expensive juicer as a used item.[18]

Choosing Your Yummy Juicing Options

Each time I fill a big bowl with fruits and vegetables and walk toward the juicer, my family just grins. I have many books on what to put into a juice, but I rarely bother. Those books have no idea where you

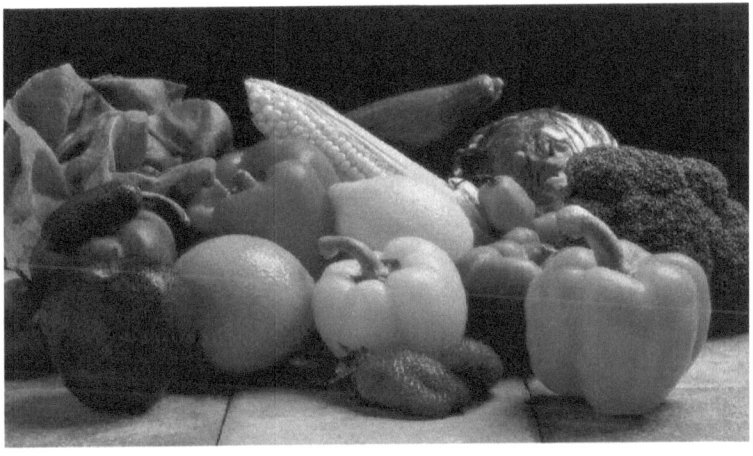

live or what fruit is in season in that geographic area. My focus is on fresh produce, well cleaned, and drinking it right away. Nothing can taste any better than the freshest of raw foods.

However, consider that fresh, raw juices will not always taste the same. Each juice is a unique opportunity to consider your individual taste preferences, what fruit is local, what time of the year makes a difference regarding if the harvest is local or a hot house item. The taste will likely be richer if it is organic, but maybe not. Are you blending for flavor or health reasons? Maybe add some ginger, garlic or basil for spiciness or health. If the weather is hot, try cucumber, carrots, or bok choy to cool down your body.

Apple is almost always a good choice with other fruits or vegetables; it is flavor neutral and therefore is often a juicing favorite. If something sweeter is required, but you are seeking a mild taste, try grapes. If you freeze the grapes first you add a chilling effect without diluting the juice with ice cubes. Another fruit that is good frozen is bananas.

Naturally, you will want to avoid overdoing very strong flavors like garlic, cabbage, and cauliflower. Also, be cautious with beets unless constipation is a current problem for which you are seeking a solution.

Beets are also high sugar, like carrots, potatoes, and parsnips. Keep in mind that vegetables grown below the ground are often sweeter.

When at all possible, chose the freshest organic fruits and vegetables you can find. The best produce going into the juicer will give the most attractive, healthiest, and best tasting output. Keep in mind that the fiber can be used right away or frozen. The extracted fiber is great for making dehydrated crackers, hot or cold soups, feed for non-carnivorous domestic animals like chickens, ducks or rabbits, and compost for enriching your soil.

Adding Health Into the Juicer

Drink your way to health. Although a broccoli, celery, tomato, garlic, ginger, and cucumber smoothie may have little appeal for breakfast, it might be just the right combination for lunch or an afternoon snack!

Let us take a closer look at juicing for health and weight control. Cancer fighters and preventatives include the berries, the cabbage family, beans and nuts. Alice Bender, a registered dietitian with the

American Institute for Cancer Research was quoted recently as saying:

> "We know that we can prevent about a third of all cancers if people would maintain a healthy weight, eat a plant-based diet, and be physically active."

The same source quoted Yikyung Park, a National Cancer Institute researcher, as stating:

> "Men and women who consumed the highest amount of dietary fiber were less likely to die from any cause." [19]

Studies have found fresh berries to be super-charged cancer fighters. Berries are an easy additive to a juicer, but keep in mind not to overdo fruits. There are chances of experiencing blood sugar imbalances if the entire day is focused on fruit. The best options are predominately fruit juice in the mornings and for one snack small drink; the rest of the day will be best made up of vegetable juices. When preparing your vegetable juices, keep dark green and leafy in mind. Adapt to so much green a little at a time to allow your digestive system and your pallet to adapt to both the type of food and the taste.

Hidden Healing Choices – Pollen and Seeds!

I have never forgotten being told that using

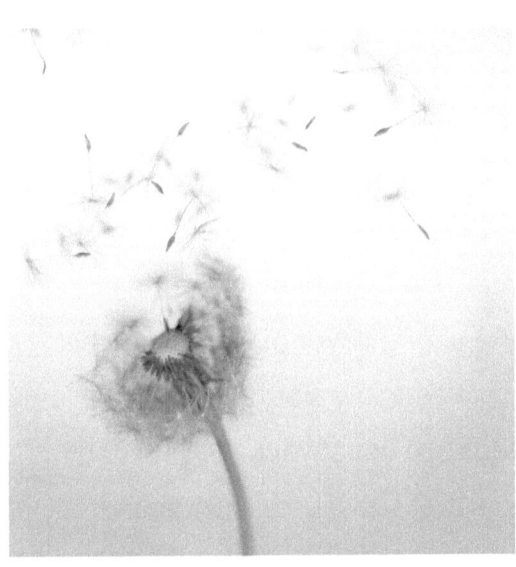

natural raw honey gathered nearby your home and used like a medicine, taking an unheated tablespoon a day, will often cure allergies. The local pollen is slowly and slightly ingested into your body from the raw (unheated) honey, like having a vaccination. That said to me that many other health options exist related to eating raw, natural, unadulterated plants. Although most vegans do not eat honey, vegetarians do. Therefore, those who suffer from allergies might try this option instead of medication.

The seeds of many fruits or vegetable add antioxidants, fiber, and other valuable natural healing properties that are typically thrown away. When juicing, tossing out part of the fruit or vegetable is not necessary. With the help of a capable masticating juicer or super high-powered blender, seeds just become a part of the smoothie. This is a means to turn an ordinary smoothie into a workhorse power drink!

Although hard to process, even the enormous avocado seed is an excellent addition to your diet. Keep in mind that the strong flavor of seeds may be difficult to adapt to, but certainly worth the effort. The treasures inside seeds are not always easy to identify, unlike package labels that say "sugar, hydrogenated oil, …" there are subtle items, like phytoestrogens, in seeds that reduce the risk of cancer by up to 40 percent.[20]

> "The total antioxidant capacity and phenolic content of edible portions and seeds of avocado, jackfruit, longan, mango and tamarind were studied. In addition, the relationship between antioxidant activity, phenolic content and the different degrees of heating of mango seed kernel was investigated. The seeds showed a much higher antioxidant activity and phenolic content than the edible portions."[21]

What Can I Juice From the Wild?

If you have been paying attention to articles about which vitamins and minerals are present in modern foods, then you are painfully aware of the loss of nutrients due to modern commercial farming methods. The continuously farmed soil has lost nutrients. Chemical fertilizer takes even more out of the soil by means of a harsh drying effect that is not enriching to the soil or the plants being grown. Many plants are harvested before maturity to enable the produce to travel long distances before being over-ripe. Some plants are "gassed" to change the color, when they are actually in a natural green state of their lifespan. The product is not mature and not actually ready for healthy eating.

All of this hardship to produce, and loss of vitality for your body, is avoided if you harvest and eat your own wild foods. The soil is naturally rich, no chemicals have been added, and there is no extensive time lapse to transport it to your home. Raw juicers seem to agree that wild grass and other eatable wild foods have higher chlorophyll contents, and are therefore, healthier than commercially raised options.

"Green leafy vegetables" is a phrase related to the most nutritious options for any human seeking weight maintenance and/or improved health. There is no saturated fat in green leafy vegetables, just Omega-3 "good fats" in small quantities. Wild grasses, stinging nettles, and dandelions are commonly known as safe wild foods to add to your juicer. Experts say that all grass is eatable. However, it is advisable to keep it 6" long or shorter as it can become bitter as it ages. Keep in mid that many juicers cannot handle grasses, even homegrown wheatgrass.

Other free food options are white pine needles, dead-nettle, flax seed micro greens, wild mint, cress, wood sorrel, purslane, henbit, wild mustard, chickweed, wild garlic mustard, wild onion, eatable flowers, wild strawberries, blackberries or blueberries, sow nettle, lambs quarters, greater plantains, clovers, daisies, and wild garlic leaves. There is a vast array of opportunities for adventuresome juicers to grab a guide (a local knowledgeable person and /or a book) and verify what might be a free nutritious meal outside your back door or down the block.

What Can I NOT Juice?

There is not enough liquid content in several eatable plants. If you are making a smoothie, not a juice, the banana is a good choice. You can add a banana to a blender and put in fresh juice with a great outcome, but you cannot juice a **banana**!

The same is true of **avocados**. If you make a fresh vegetable juice, you can add a fresh, pealed avocado to the blender and pour in the fresh juice for a smoothie, but you cannot juice an avocado!

Even after the extremely hard outside shell is removed, the **coconut** "meat" (the firm part of the inside of the coconut) is typically too hard to juice and lacking enough liquid. You can blend some varieties of the coconut meat with the milk (the liquid inside the coconut) for a smoothie.

In the onion family, the mature **leek** looks like a scallion on steroids! They are huge, have an extremely strong flavor, and have very little juice. Additionally, they are very hard on juicers.

Looking like colored celery, **rhubarb** can grow very large. It is a very tough vegetable that can break juicers. It has very effective laxative qualities.

Finally, **winter squash** is considered not juicable. The outside skin is extremely hard; it may ruin a juicer.

Juicing Avoids Harmful, Hidden GMO Mutations

Making your own fresh juice as an avenue to weight loss and health has a significant advantage over powdered or ready-to-drink processed weight loss foods. Many processed foods contain chemical additives that have been shown to cause illnesses in humans, pigs, cows and rats. These additives or genetically modified (GM) organisms (GMO) are not listed as such on the labels in the USA. The unknowing consumer is causing harm to his or her self without having a means to avoid it unless you travel to Europe where all GMO products are for good reasons, banned. Eating fresh, organic foods, like home squeezed juices, completely avoids those dangers even in the USA and other countries where GMO's are allowed.

What is a GMO? A GM or GMO is a way to introduce bacterial genes into corn, soy, or other plants 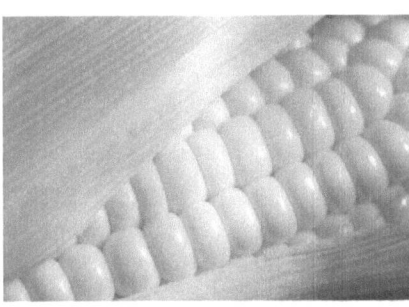 to make certain they continue to thrive after being sprayed with herbicide. An herbicide is a product that normally kills a plant. Some of these GM modified plants produce a poison that is created within the plant to increase resistance to disease. The human or animal that eats the plant or a processed portion of the food product also eats the dangerous chemical. GMO treated soy is often used in infant formulas and nearly 70% of all processed foods.[22] Unbiased studies have found various dangers from eating GM treated plants.

How are genetically modified organisms a real danger to humans?

"It appears there is a direct correlation between GMOs and autism." --Arden Anderson, MD, PhD, MPH[23]

In 2009, the American Academy of Environmental Medicine (AAEM) stated that, "Several animal studies indicate serious health risks associated with genetically modified (GM) food," including infertility, immune problems, accelerated aging, faulty insulin regulation, and changes in major organs and the gastrointestinal system. The AAEM has asked physicians to advise all patients to avoid GM foods.[24]

There is a free guide to enable the consumer to completely avoid GMO laced foods.[25] Consider learning more about this problem to prevent or cure diseases in those you know and love.

"Mainstream medicine would be way different if they focused on prevention even half as much as they focused on intervention..."

~Anonymous

Chapter Three - Appreciate Your Glowing Slender Health

"The greatest wealth is health.

Just because you're not sick doesn't mean you're healthy"

~Author Unknown

Realistically Defining Your Goals

Although you have already decided that losing weight is the goal you want to achieve. You my not have clearly defined how you will do that using a juice fast. So, before you begin fasting on juice find out who you are so that the goals you set are realistic to your abilities, personality, needs, wants, and what will drive you to success. Do a self-assessment by taking an unbiased look at YOU.

Free psychological tests are available online that will help you to have a better understanding of yourself. Most are abridged since you are a layperson taking a test that is normally given and interpreted by a professional. These self-tests are helpful, but not perfect. Use them as a guide to where you might need to go to get more help to meet your goals.

The Myers-Briggs test is in the book titled "Please Understand Me." The greatest understanding you will receive is about you! Try the Myers-Briggs Type Indicator Assessment.[26] More than any other test; the Myers-Briggs has helped many to understand where he or she fits, out of sixteen personality types. It will help you to understand why you act like you do. Wouldn't you also like to have that information?

There are several other self-help tests. For example, the Strong-Campbell Interest Inventory[27] is an assessment that takes the answers to questions of people in certain professions and matches those with your replies to the exact same questions to see if any of those professions would be a good choice for you. You can even assess for mental health personality types. Mental wellness is a few degrees away from mental illness. It is good to understand what makes you who you are, so go online and take the MMPI.[28] The results will not make any sense to you. There are no "right" or "wrong" answers to 567 questions answered in 90 minutes. An advance reading of the questions to make sure you understand them does not harm this true/false test. You will need a professional to do the analysis and explain the results.

You will know:

- who you are,
- how you typically analyze things,
- what drives you,
- when you get motivated,
- where you want to go,
- and some more interesting facts.

This is the information you need to take charge of

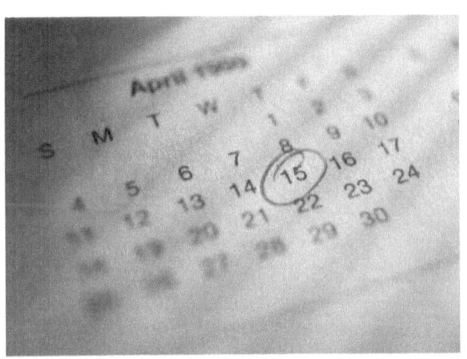

your future by taking an action – creating goals - that will put you in control. A goal is a measurable outcome that allows you to define a desirable end. Normally, you work hard to reach it through a series of calculated (or chance) steps. There you will see clearly how you are progressing. At last, you will verify success.

Each goal must be:

S = significant	and/or	specific
M = meaningful	and/or	measurable
A = action oriented	and/or	attainable
R = reliant	and/or	rewarding
T = time	and/or	trackable

Each goal you define must have <u>all of these attributes</u>.

Examples:

Very Short Term Weight Loss Goal for anyone: *Today, I will drink 6-8 glasses of water, make three glasses of veggie juice and one of fruits juice. I imagine that each glass is entering my body as a natural cleanse that is making me healthier than I have ever thought possible.*

Very Short Term Weight Loss Goal for a caregiver of other family members: *This morning I feel like my will power is very high, no matter how much solid food smells or looks good to me, I know that to focus on making the freshest and most delicious juice is the best option for me today. By evening I will feel even stronger* and better able to care for my family's needs, and yet, stay on my detox program.

Very Short Term Weight Loss Goal for a caregiver of friends: *Today, my weight continues to move toward the healthiest level for me. Although I am on this pathway of detoxing all alone, I know that soon my friends will join me, within a month, in getting back our slim inner selves. This is my time to work on becoming a mentor to others who have followed the out-of-control roadway to weight gain. We will overcome this obstacle!*

Short Term Weight Loss Goal: *On Friday, I will make sure I have all my eating for the day done by 6pm so that I can relax on the couch until 11 pm without eating as I watch TV.*

Medium Term Weight Loss Goal: *Before December 15, of this year I will lose 34 pounds so that I can wear my aunt's 40-year old wedding dress for my own wedding*

Long Term Weight Loss Goal: *Within ten years I will wear a size 6 dress, jeans, and coat as my own choice to look as young as I feel.*

In most cases goal setting can be short term or long term. However, it is a really good idea to have many short-term goals at the beginning of a weight loss program. Make each goal only slightly longer than the last, to keep motivated. Make certain that any reward during the entire process is not food related. Make sure all terms are understandable early on in the process and consistent during the entire process.

Very Short Term Goals are something accomplished within hours or one day:

- I will take this bowl of colorful veggies and make the best juice I have ever tasted to enable my body to transform into a sexy, "feel great" shape.

Short Term Goals are something accomplished within six months or one year:

- I will take a **logic** test and better understand how I would be best motivated to focus my energies using logic for weight loss.

Medium Term Goals are something accomplished typically in more than one and less than five years.

- I will **purchase** a size 10 dress and plan to wear it in eighteen months to my best friend's wedding due to losing excess weight consistently and exercising every day until then.

Long Term Goals are something accomplished typically in more than five, but not much more than ten years.

- I will develop **a new lifestyle** of juice fasting for 4 days every month after I get down to a size 6 as that will enable me to keep that size for the rest of my life.

Post your goals in places where you will see them every day, more than once a day. Read them out loud first thing every morning and last thing every night.

Writing Your Own Success Story

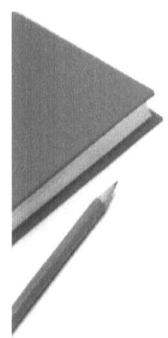

Start keeping a journal as soon as you have made the commitment to juice fast for weight loss. You might even want to write a blog. However, a public statement each day might be too personal for you. Evaluate your own personality by beginning the journal first, and simply taking the pieces out of it that would be good in a blog.

Another helpful tool is to join an online juice fasting support group. There are many to choose from, so look around until you find one that has people you feel "at home" talking to. Make sure you are both realistic and visionary. Do not allow one naysayer to draw you away from your goals. Say your own goals every morning, and again right before you go on the blog so that you are at your own emotional high point as you inner the fasting support group. Using a fasting support group might be an outstanding way to prepare you for mentoring your friends toward this same self-empowering means to weight loss.

It took time to pack on the pounds; it will take time to take them off. Some days an entire pound will exit your body; other days you will plateau. Regardless of how quickly or slowly you body is willing to give up excess weight, know that every day you are getting healthier. The price of health cannot be measured in money spent. The value of health is measured in years enjoyed.

Pack your years with the joy of wearing clothing that is not getting too tight to wear comfortably. Imagine how much fun clothing shopping will be when you have the shape that designers use to make new clothing styles. It is totally amazing to realize that your story will always have a happy ending as long as you continue to enjoy a variety of fresh vegetable juices every day. You cannot fail if you simply stick to drinking a variety of fresh juices each time you are hungry or feeling the need for more energy. This is not a career challenge that can have many outcomes. This is a simple math problem solved:

Glasses of spring water + glasses of freshly squeezed juices = weight loss

As you write your own unique story, be sure to address how you feel each day. Keep a record of your highs and lows. Make every effort to stay "in touch" with what is happening to you.

- Did you exercise to speed along your weight loss or toning?
- Did you begin walking outdoors to both tone your body and take healing energy from simply being in nature?
- Did you read more?
- Did you watch TV less or more?
- What did your friends say to you?
- What did you enjoy the most?
- What did you fear the most?
- How will you behave differently next time?
- Did you add more goals as you went along?
- Any really weird things occur?

Relating to the "really weird thing" is the story of a gal who was determined to fast on only water until her hunger returned. The time was the early 1970's, and it her first extended fast. At the time, most literature on fasting was written in the 1940's. Very little was written about healing with fasting; most was recording fasting for spiritual reasons. She had suffered for years with ulcerative colitis and had been told that water fasting gives the colon an opportunity to heal as the bowels totally empty. She decided to try water fasting and see what results occurred.

All was going well as she entered the 16th night. As she laid her head on her pillow, with her right ear down and her head and body pointing toward her right side, her left tear duct began to drain pus down her cheek. For what seemed like an eternity, that pus ran down her cheek. Rather than panic, she thought about what an amazing sign her body was giving her that some old infection was now finally able to leave her body. She had read that when no effort is being made to digest food, the body has an opportunity to focus on the elimination of toxins. This was her proof!

At the end of her 21 days fast, she had lost 28 pounds of excess fat. Following the books she read very carefully, she had a tablespoon of fresh squeezed orange juice every 15 minutes for four hours and only raw foods for the next week. She kept the weight off and her colon was much improved, but it was the pus coming from her tear duct that left the longest impression. Her body had given her an unexpected, unique sign that fasting was a great opportunity for healing. She continued to fast the rest of her life as a pathway to weight maintenance and healing.

Do not forget that every part of your own story has a great deal of value. Most people who fully experience juice fasting for weight loss will use it as a tool to keep weight off. Some fast one day a week, others three to four days every month or quarter, and still others for two weeks every six months. Your way of eating will dictate your new pattern of weight maintenance. There are those who use juice fasting as a way to move from a high-fat diet with lots of snack foods into a vegetarian or vegan diet. They may never need to fast again. Everyone is different and gets to choose for themselves. The important part is to keep your journal as a reference for the future – YOUR future. After this adventure, if you follow this plan, your self-knowledge will be at a new all time high.

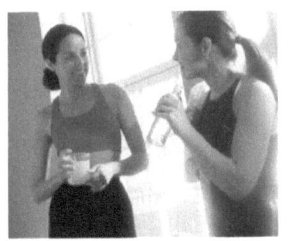

Finding Fantastic Fat-Free Flavors

The journey into a whole new world is about to begin. Although most first time juice fasters have tasted fresh-squeezed orange juice, It is likely that was the exception rather than the rule. Few places offer fresh-squeezed orange juice as a standard option. That trend has already been modified in the West: Oregon, Washington, and California. Therefore, it will change elsewhere. However, bottled juices will not outclass the value of fresh squeezed juice. Agree to give in. Buy your own juicer and use it every day! Your new, slim body will thank you.

There are so many colors, flavors, and resulting natural healing options to choose from when choosing to juice fast. Start out with apple and carrot; add green celery, cucumber, spinach, and other green leafy vegetables. "The greener the better" seems to be an on-going theme for those starting out with raw juice fasting.

Save the all fruit drinks for breakfast since too much natural sugar can interfere with blood sugar metabolism especially in those who have diabetes or hypoglycemia. After a morning glass of juice and two or three of water, settle into a day of veggie juices. If any seem too tart, add an apple or a few frozen grapes to give a little sweetness. Keep in mind that carrots are nearly always sweet; add one to any tart juice. Sugar beets are too sweet (and bowel loosening) to eat often. Melon is a great item to juice as a desert juice. It is very high in water content, tastes sweet, and yet is low calorie. The Spanish speaking culture cuts it half with water and drinks "melon water" in place of high sugar carbonated drinks. Kids love it!

Most fruit and vegetable options are fat-free. Since fat is 9 calories a gram and carbohydrates are only 4 calories a gram, it is easy to see how fat does make us fat (regardless of how often we were told otherwise before the obesity crisis became obvious and global.) Human beings enjoy the taste of sweet like breast milk and ripe berries in the spring. We have developed an acquired taste for highly processed fats in our foods. Diets that stress a very high intake of fat and protein have been found to be detrimental to health in general and the heart specifically.[29,30, 31]

Wheat grass and barley grass are outstanding in juice fasting detoxing or weight loss programs. However, many juicers are unable to handle juicing them. Check the manufacturer's instructions to see if your juicer will. Often people will put these in a blender and then add the pulverized end product into the juice.

Cayenne can be added to any fresh squeezed juice. It will increase energy, dissolve mucus, and it stops internal bleeding (intestines, uterus, etc.). Cayenne increases the movement of blood in the body so strokes and other circulation is improved using Cayenne. Take only 1/8 teaspoon of 150,000 Heat units a day and work up to more taken in the juice – never alone.

Organic, unfiltered apple cider or grape vinegar is a terrific additive for those who suffer from arthritis. Use about a teaspoon a day. If you have a cold during a fast, simply add cayenne, fresh ginger, onion, and vinegar to a veggie juice drink; allow your natural healing to begin.

Algae can be added to fresh juices for essential amino acids. The types include Spirulina, Chlorella, blue green algae, and Dunaliella (red algae). The body absorbs algae instantly with about a 70% utilization factor. Add a ½ teaspoon of the powder into your juice. It does not mix well but the powder is the best way. It is a highly nutritious food; do not allow it get too hot.

Nutritional yeast (saccharomyces cerevasiae) is another outstanding juice additive. Nutritional yeast is very high in B vitamins, including B12 (the evasive one that vegans have very few ways to obtain). It is best to begin by taking one tablespoon a day, and work up to ingesting two tablespoons daily. One authority stated the following:

> "Since nutritional yeast is so high in B vitamins, and the nervous system requires so much of them to function properly, this makes an excellent food for the brain, peripheral nerves, and spinal cord. Those with nervous system disorders such as myasthenia gravis, multiple sclerosis, brain diseases such as

Alzheimer's disease, premature senility, all types of dementia, schizophrenia, Tourette's syndrome, and other neurologic diseases may want to increase their dose as needed. People with milder neurologic problems such as anxiety, depression, mental, and emotional disorders will benefit too."[32]

Discovering Numerous Health Benefits

Not only will juice fasting reduce your body weight, but also the lack of high fat intake will help your heart. High carbohydrate and low fat diets lower your risk of having a heart attack. When juice fasting, the digestive process is very gentle as the juice is almost immediately absorbed into the body. In High fat and high protein diets, the body has to work very hard to digest the dense food.

Also, due to our very long digestive tract, the heavy proteins stay in the gut for a very long time. Some researchers believe that during that time, the body absorbs a great deal of the recombinant bovine growth hormone (rBGH), an injection that is given to cattle. Cattle injected with rBGH suffer a loss of immunity and are given many more antibiotics that also pass into the humans who drink their milk, eat cheese or meat. According to The American Cancer Society, rBGH causes illnesses in cattle. Furthermore, rBGH has been studied a great deal as having a possible link to cancer in humans who eat meat or dairy. At this time, there is no definitive conclusion.[33] Humans, who eat meat or dairy, are said by some observers to develop a resistance to the positive effects of antibiotics they need during a human illness. That is due to the overexposure of antibiotics that pass through the meat or dairy and creates a resistance in people. When needed antibiotics are offered to him or her to overcome a human disease; the disease germ in the human is not overcome.[34]

Ending Juice Fasting Correctly

The only dangers when juice fasting is not taking it slow when reintroducing solid foods. Give your digestive tract time to adapt to the changes as to not cause an upset. When the human body has been only accepting easy-to-digest fresh juices, the introduction of solid foods needs to be done slowly. Do not even think about eating processed foods!

Start with a small piece of fresh fruit or some lettuce. Chew the food a great deal. Avoid fats, like salad dressings, and use a squeeze of lemon or lime instead. Do not eat bread the first day. The first couple of days, think baby food: soft fruits, mushy vegetables, and well-cooked cereals. The longer you have fasted, the slower you need to go returning to solid foods. If you only fasted for 36 hours over a weekend, just take it easy on Monday with a light breakfast, a salad at noon, and a vegetarian dinner. If you have juice fasted for 30 days, be very careful to eat vegan lightly (no meat or dairy) for the first week before going back to your normal diet.

Choosing Permanent Weight Loss

If your main reason for fasting was to loose weight, then going back to your "normal" diet is not going to keep it off. This is a perfect time to make some definitive choices related to a lifetime change. You can certainly choose to juice fast as is needed to get your

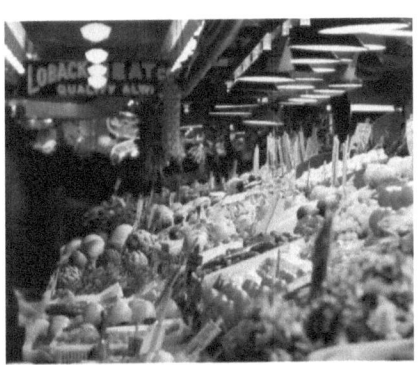 weight back to where you want it to be. You can get yourself on a schedule of so many days a week, month, or year.

Another option is a lifestyle change. There are many pathways to follow that will help keep the weight off. Here are a few examples:

Raw food – 75% raw food (not heated over 115 degrees f)

Vegan – no flesh, dairy or animal products (no eggs, honey or lard); avoids most processed foods not labeled "Vegan" or "Organic." This is often termed a "lifestyle" as deep ecologists often choose this option.

Fat-free Vegan – all of vegan and no added vegetable oils

Lacto – Vegetarian – no animal flesh: no beef, pork, poultry, fish, eggs or shellfish, but do eat dairy.

Lacto – Ovo - Vegetarian – no animal flesh: no beef, pork, poultry, fish or shellfish, but do eat eggs and dairy.

Ovo-Vegetarian - no animal flesh: no beef, pork, poultry, dairy, milk, fish or shellfish, but does eat eggs.

Pescatarian – no animal flesh other than fish

Pollo – vegetarian - no animal flesh other than chicken

Macrobiotic – unprocessed vegan foods, avoids sugar and oils, some fish, lots of Asian vegetables.

Fruitarian – eats only fruits (that includes tomatoes, eggplant, zucchini, avocadoes, seeds, and nuts).

Flexitarian – follows a lacto-ovo vegetarian path but has animal flesh occasionally.

Chapter Four - Enjoy Your Fitness Rebound

"Those who think they have no time for exercise will sooner or later have to find time for illness."
~Edward Stanley

Getting to Know the New You

This aspect of using juice fasting is a lot harder than you can imagine. If a lot of time has passed with your body being a size larger than when you were in high school, you have probably adapted to that new size. You may even have forgotten what the old you felt like. This chapter describes what that statement means, how I found the body I had as the old me, and what I did, and continue to do, to keep it slender.

I began fasting in 1976, three years before I became a vegetarian. However, it was not until many years later that I discovered the advantages of juice fasting, a fat-free detox that helped me manage my weight and had numerous additional health benefits. For most of those years without meat in my life, I was vegetarian, not vegan. Therefore, I ate dairy. I was kidding myself that I had the answer to health with that diet; dairy is a killer. Dairy may actually be far worse than meat, but then I did not know that. Now you do! Honestly, it was not until I gave up dairy, and all added fats, that I really started to live in absolute joy with the body I had always wanted. The feeling is something I struggle to describe to you now, because it was so unimaginable to the old me. I felt trapped in my fat thighs that rubbed together all the time. It was so hard to love me, when I hated those wobbly, rubbing thighs so much.

Connecting With Your Inner Self

If I was going to win at the weight loss game, I thought I would look at what the experts were doing. Like Ali Vincent, the first female to win "The Biggest Loser," I had always used a wide variety of physical exercises, with and without various pieces of equipment, and "good" eating to manage my weight. However, like most very active people, I often had aches and pains that prevented my exercising enough to keep the weight off. Additionally, life got in the way with work or school deadlines, ill family members, obligations for my charity or just a flat tire. It was always something!

I watched videos of Ali Vincent and realized that she was working out an excessive amount and yet, her thighs still rubbed together! Therefore, I finally realized that exercise and "good" eating was just not enough to give me the body I wanted and to maintain the body I wanted. This hit me again when I read Jillian Michaels book, "Making the Cut."[35] She said something about preparing for a big sports event and being in perfect shape. However, that was not a place that could always be maintained. She complained in 2012 about bringing two children into her family within two weeks. Therefore, she had avoided the gym for just two weeks, and she was loosing her shape. Gads! Chris Crowley and Dr. Henry Lodge offered me the same message in "Younger Next Year," to stay active and stay slim.[36] Stop being active, day-after-day, and get fat again right away.

I thought, Whoa! That may be true for an athlete, but as a woman, a wife, a mother, and a professional, I wanted to get thinner and stay that way. I wanted to wear one wardrobe day-after-day without such extreme physical effort based on me not hurting myself during exercise. Not losing the weight loss game due to a week or two without extreme exercise being undertaken. In looking around, it seemed not. Most people I knew were overweight, a great deal overweight. Many of my closest friends are clinically obese. Were there really any answers out there?

Adding More Lifestyle Changes

Not being the type of person to give up, I began to look further. Because I totally believe in natural healing, and scientific facts, I started looking at "The Father of Medicine." His oath is still used today when anyone becomes a physician. He must have had some pretty insightful theories. I found this quote and realized that concept had been my pathway since high school. Continuing to follow it made sense, but what food would be my medicine?

"Let food be thy medicine and medicine be thy food"

~ Hippocrates (431 B.C.E.)

In the same way that reading one true story, "Many Lives, Many Masters" by a highly respected psychiatrist Brian L. Weiss, helped me to bridge the gap between medicine and psychiatric insight; I found other medical scientists who were not afraid to report their findings. I did that by focusing first on health and second on weight loss and maintenance. It was while on this journey that I found many answers.[37,38,39,40]

Apparently, the world was not ready for "The China Study" when it was published in 2006.[37] Perhaps now that more people around the globe have passed the mark on a weight scale that makes them dangerously overweight, they will listen. In 2013, predictions include more people embracing a plant-based diet.[41]

Juice fasting is embracing a raw, fat-free liquid nearly predigested (optionally organic) vegan diet. Most readers will accept this option for a period of time; others will feel like they have found the Holy Grail. I fell "crashing" into the second group. I realized that by eating more raw organic juices, I was getting vitamins, minerals, and other nutrients that we not available anywhere else. I was training my mind to be satisfied with a glass of juice as lunch. If you can also feel that way, it is possible to substitute fresh juice for a meal throughout your week, like a mini fast.

It may be possible for you to create a habit of ingesting juice or raw foods more frequently.

Fortunately for me, I had been happy with just a salad and lemon juice topping for a very long time. I grew up on meat no more than twice a week, fish we caught ourselves, and an occasional chicken that Dad and I raised. Most of my childhood meals were vegetarian. The leap into raw juices or vegan meals is much harder for those who have been used to eating about 1,000 calories in a single child's "Happy Meal"[42] or 1,844 calories and 103 grams for fat for the adult portion of a fast path to a heart attack.[43] Juice fasting is a healthy, natural way to reverse that trend, lose weight, and get healthier.

Maintaining Your New Shape

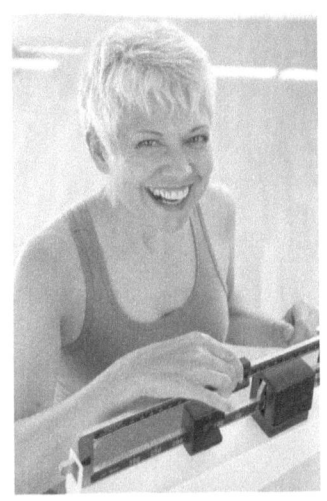

Regardless of how long you juice fast to lose weight, trading 2,200 calories or more a day that is filled with fat for fat-free juice will result in significant weight loss over a short and long period of time.

Some people, who have stored a considerable amount more than their frame was met to carry, might lose a pound a day when juice fasting. The real win is to not only to lose the weight but also, to keep it off.

If you think that after a few days of drinking only raw, fat-free fresh juices, you body is going to maintain the same low weight on 1,844 calorie third meals of the day, then you probably do not clearly understand the principals of weight loss. When drinking only raw, fat-free fresh juices, you are taking in nearly predigested nutrients that your body puts right to work healing you. As soon as you begin to be actively moving and requiring energy to feed your muscles, your body reaches for stored fat and burns it for energy; you lose weight. If instead you use up only 1,500 calories a day being active, and eat 2,800 calories a day, the extra 1,300 calories are stored as fat; you gain weight.

Therefore, if you have lost the weight and want to keep it off you need to take in each day only what you are using up. You already know that you need fewer calories than you did in the past when you were gaining weight. What you need is a new lifestyle.

- You can choose to augment your previous eating patterns with periods of juice fasting.
- You might like to highly increase your activity level.
- Maybe you would rather skip some solid food meals and replace them with fresh juice.
- Otherwise you can try switching to a plant-based diet, and rarely have to be concerned about maintaining your weight.

Regardless of your choice, be sure to settle on a choice before you stop juice fasting. Yo-yo dieting, and then gaining a great deal of weight, is not the best option for your health. Most experts suggest staying within a two-pound range.

Mentoring Another to Find Joy

After juice fasting has given you the body you always dreamed of having, do not expect your friends to come running to you to find out how you lost so much weight. Most modern adults are looking for a quick fix to remove weight and without any hassle. The idea of buying a juicer and fresh items to juice each day is not likely to appeal to them. Even when you tell them about how good it feels to fit into old clothing or to buy a new wardrobe. All of your comments will fall on deaf ears until they **decide** that they are ready to lose weight. Some people are motivated by laboratory reports or a doctor's bad news about a test result. Seeing him or her self in a photo next to a former classmate or a spouse motivates a few people. Other people are triggered when a relative dies of an environmentally imposed disease. Whatever motivates anyone will need to come from within themselves. Your job is to be ready to help when they ask and not before.

After your friend has the same results as you have had, then being motivators for each other is a great help in staying on track. It is also fun to share maintenance ideas, recipes, and exercise events.

Chapter Five - Living a Life of Quality and Vitality

"In order to change, we must be sick and tired of being sick and tired."

~Author Unknown

Finding Self Expression Using The 3 C's!

To successfully lose weight by juice fasting you need just three C's: Courage, Compassion, and Connection. First, you need the Courage to begin, and then carry out the juice fast to the end. Second, you need the Compassion to acknowledge that you are human. You may slip and fall, but you can always start again, and be successful. Finally, you need the Connection with all the tools offered to help you. Friends, relatives, online support groups, articles, books, personal trainers or whatever else it takes to reach your weight goal.

Just about anything we do in life, we do because we think it will be better than what we had before we did it. That is how we find the courage. We marry because we do not want to face life alone. We become parents because we want a family of our own or others pressure us into choosing that option to please them. We divorce because the union did not work out like we had imagined it should have been. We recover from abuse of our bodies due to smoking, self-medication, excess alcohol, over-eating, gambling or other vice because it seems appropriate for others or ourselves. We move to another geographic location or residence because it seems like that place might make us happier, feel more secure, look of a higher social status, or some other emotional reason. We face an empty nest because we chose to not give birth to or adopt/foster more children. We retire due to feeling like that would be better than working at what was available for us for an income.

Sometimes we have no real option. We deal with a loss or trauma because we often have no choice. We work at a soul-leaching job because it is all we have been able to acquire. We have an empty bank account because where the money went was a necessity or out of your control.

We acknowledge the need to show compassion for our feelings. Making the decision to lose weight is often due to feeling like the pain of denial is better than the shame and discomfort of carrying around your lovely self inside so much hampering bulk. Perhaps, we made the decision to lose weight because of medical advice or to avoid dealing with bias or bullying. In any case, at some point we choose to make an effort for a very good reason.

The next step is to have others develop an emotional supportive attitude, a connection to us, and our goals. Preventing them or you from sabotaging your plans is a difficult next move. This is nothing new as the following quote points out.

"Our bodies are our gardens – our wills are our gardeners."

~William Shakespeare

Be very clear that saying "just this once" and eating something is what made you overweight in the first place. Decide what you are going to do, and do it.

Every single time you slip backwards, get up, brush yourself off and get right back on track regardless of what else is going on. When you meet your weight goal, be very clear about how you are going to stay slim. Love the new you. Praise your looks, your ease of movements, and what you can do more than you ever imagined that you could. Do not allow yourself to go back to you came from again. You are a winner!

Branching Out Without Bias

In the process of loving you, it is not necessary to dislike anyone else. If your friends become former friends because you have decided to put you first, they were not true friends. If other makes catty remarks about you "Dressing like a person half your age," acknowledge that it is fun to be able to wear youthful clothing, but do not fall into the trap being set for you to fail. You are being asked to get fat again and be "One of the gang," because the speakers do not want to go to the effort to accomplish what you have done.

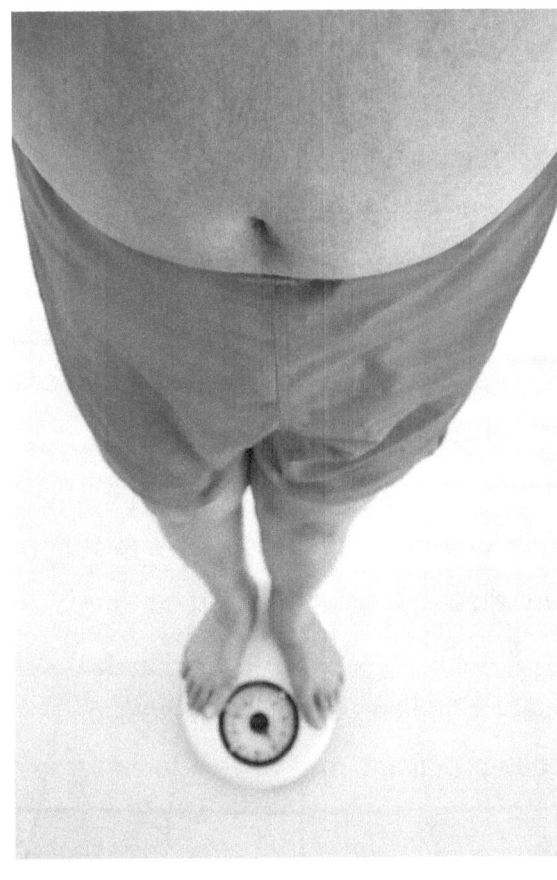

Take responsibility for your weight and your health, every day, regardless of where you are or what you are doing. You ARE worth the effort! Eating greasy French fries with other people, when two in the room have diagnosed heart disease, is not being loving toward each participant. Entering the room with a lovely bowl of fruit is a loving act. The others do not have to eat it, but they have the option because you brought it. You also have the healthier food option, and do not have the "excuse" that the only thing to eat was the greasy French fries.

You are human. You can slip anytime. Be humbly grateful that you lost the weight, but do not act arrogant. You know the secret, juice fasting, share it when asked. Use it to stay thin.

Exploring Life as a Slender Adult

There are many things that you can do now that you would not do when you were physically larger. For example, when Ali Vincent was 234 pounds she appeared burdened and sluggish. At 125 pounds, she was smiling and perky. At her first weight, she might not have been able to win a job that she would be more likely to get at her second weight. Bias against overweight people not "looking good" in the position or fear of higher health premiums may have kept her from getting a job.

Overweight people are naturally tired and, generally, do not get as much done by carrying around the additional weight. That extra 50 or 100 pounds is a real burden. A dear friend noticed this in his business. He ran a motel. He said that he could not recall a time when clinically obese people came in and the room was not totally trashed. The effort to pick up a towel and hang it on a shower rod might be just too much to ask.

Therefore losing weight might open an entire new side of your life. Maybe you will start an online business, become a model, go into sales, become a travel agent, and number of jobs that require the high energy that can be acquired only after ridding your body of that additional heavy burden that was always there.

Looking Youthful and Feeling Fit
The following words are generally not in the vocabulary of a person who is clinically obese.

- Bikini shopping
- Little black dress
- Feeling really sexy
- In a crowd, eyes turn toward your entrance
- A perfect blind date choice
- Let's go for a l-o-n-g walk
- I love tennis! (or any other active sport)
- Really? I'd have guessed you 10 years younger

- Let's take an adventure vacation

However, all of the above are normal comments for those having mastered and maintained their weight loss goals.

The following words are generally often in the report of a medical doctor who just examined a person who is clinically obese.

- Your blood pressure is too high
- You are on the verge of diabetes
- Your heart is straining under your current weight
- I am concerned about your kidney function
- You are going to need knee or hip replacement surgery soon
- Your arches are severely broken down
- Operating is very risky at your weight
- Your family history of cancer related to obesity puts you at a higher risk

The choice of being in the first or second group really is yours. Juice fasting is your easiest healthy option.

Chapter Six - Exploring Some Juicing Recipes

Plain and Simple

Juicing is a fun process with a great deal of room for creativity. Do not hesitate to try new things. Keep in mind that the amount of liquid in a piece of fruit or vegetable and the size of either can vary a great deal. You can always add a little water or set some apple or carrot juice aside to add to any other juice. Do not be afraid to experiment with whatever is ripe in your area. You might find some very special combinations.

Carrot Apple Delight
Juice 4 carrots to 1 apple

Carrot Orange Joy
Juice 4 carrots to 1 orange

Illness Specific
Start with: Carrot Apple Delight - Juice 4 carrots to 1 apple

Overweight? Add some citrus

Restless or Depressed? Add some celery

Diabetes? Reduce to 2 carrots; then add some celery, parsley, cucumber, and/or garlic

Kidney or prostrate disorders? Add horseradish

Infections? Colds? Flu? Add lemons, oranges, pineapple, berries, beets, greens

Stomach problems? Add celery, tomatoes, cabbage, grapes, beets

Losing your hair? Take a handful of alfalfa sprouts, 4/5 leaves of fresh lettuce, one whole lemon and one cucumber.
Wrinkle on skin? Again take one lemon, one cucumber, a handful of watercress, two large carrots and some ginger root.

Green Lighting

Green Meany

Juice 2 carrots, 2 apples, ½ a beet, 2 broccoli florets, a stalk of chard or spinach, a pinch of parsley, cilantro, or basil, ½ a lemon or orange! Add more leafy greens as you adapt to the taste.

Desert Green

Juice 2 apples, 2 carrots, ½ a pineapple stick, 2 pad of Napoli cactus, a stalk of chard or spinach, a pinch of parsley, cilantro, or basil, ½ a lemon or orange!

Meal Specific
Breakfast:

Carrot Soylicious

Juice 4 carrots to ½ -1 cup of soymilk (hemp, oat or almond will work)

Optional nutmeg, mace, or cinnamon on top

Berry DayBreak

Juice 3 apples, 1 pear and a handful of berries (frozen is fine)

Lunch or Dinner:

Carrot Tomlicious

Juice 3 carrots to ½ a beet, 2 tomatoes, and two stick of celery with leaves – if you have some fresh basil, add a pinch!

Carrot Spice

Juice 5 carrots, 1 clove of fresh garlic, and 4 stick of celery with leaves - chili, add a pinch!

Apple Snap!

Juice 3 apples, 1 lemon or lime, ½" slice of fresh ginger

Beet Energy Drop

Juice 4 carrots, 1-2 apples, 1 beet with tops, and ½ a cucumber – if you have trouble relaxing add a stick or two of celery

5 helpful Tips about Juicing.

* Try to mix as much as green vegetable as your taste bud can handle (specially greens such as Kale, broccoli, spinach and other leafy greens)

* Add some ginger root as it has many health benefits and it also helps reduce the bitterness in some green juice.

* To increase amount of juice, you can always add more cucumber to any juice without altering the taste.

* If you are diabetic, try to limit your intake of sweet fruits and sweet vegetables like carrots.

* Try to add some type berries (even frozen) into your juicing practice.

References

1. http://healthland.time.com/2009/07/31/american-spending-on-yoga-echinacea-and-acupuncture/
2. Airola, Paavo, 1971. *Juice Fasting,* The Age-Old Way to a New You. Health Plus Publishers, Sherwood, Oregon, USA.
3. Ozersky, Josh, 2012. Big Gulp. Time Magazine 3/12/2012, Vol. 179 Issue 10, p112-113.
4. http://online.wsj.com/article/SB10001424052970204358004577030112155716538.html/
5. http://money.cnn.com/2011/01/05/news/companies/starbucks_new_logo/index.htm
6. Pathy, R; Mills, K. E.; Gazeley, S.; Ridgley, A.; Kiran, T., 2011. Health is a spiritual thing: perspectives of health care professionals and female Somali and Bangladeshi women on the health impacts of fasting during Ramadan. *Ethnicity & Health.* Feb2011, Vol. 16 Issue 1, p43-56.
7. Imai S. SIRT1 and caloric restriction: an insight into possible trade-offs between robustness and frailty. Curr Opin Clin Nutr Metab Care. 2009;12:350–356. doi: 10.1097/MCO.0b013e32832c932d.
8. Vaquero A, Reinberg D. Calorie restriction and the exercise of chromatin. Genes Dev. 2009;23:1849–1869. doi: 10.1101/gad.1807009.
9. Anson, R.M., Guo, Z., Rafael de Cabo, Iyun, T., Rios, M., Hagepanos, A., Ingram, D.K., Lane, M.A., & Mattson, M. P., 2002. Intermittent fasting dissociates beneficial effects of dietary restriction on glucose metabolism and neuronal resistance to injury from calorie intake. National Academy of Sciences. Internet retrieved Nov., 22, 2012 from http://www.pnas.org.
10. Trepanowski, J.F., Canale, R.E., Marshall, K.E., Kabir, M.M., Bloomer, R.J., 2011. Impact of caloric and dietary restriction regimens on markers of health and longevity in humans and animals: a summary of available findings. Bio Med Central Ltd. *Nutritional Journal,* 10:107.
11. http://www.dailymail.co.uk/health/article-2098363/Fasting-help-combat-cancer-boost-effectiveness-treatments.html
12. http://www.freedomyou.com/fasting__healed_of_ovarian_cancer_freedomyou.aspx
13. Bishop, Beata. A Time to Heal. England.
14. http://gerson.org/gerpress/dr-max-gerson/

15. http://www.allergyreliefexpert.com/fasting-for-allergies/
16. http://blueprintcleanse.com/experts-opinion.html
17. http://www.fernsnutrition.com/juicers.html
18. http://www.discountjuicers.com/classifieds/view.cgi
19. Elizabeth Agnvall, 2012. Eat to Prevent Cancer. AARP Bulletin, December 2012, pg. 12 – 16.
20. http://www.dailymail.co.uk/health/article-2037255/Breast-cancer-Eating-flaxseeds-reduce-risk-dying-40-cent.html
21. Yean-Yean Soong and Phillip J. Barlow, 2004. Antioxidant activity and phenolic content of selected fruit seeds. *□ood □he□istry,* Vol. 88: 3, pgs. 411-417.
22. http://www.responsibletechnology.org/consumers
23. http://www.responsibletechnology.org/autism
24. http://www.aaemonline.org/gmopost.html
25. http://responsibletechnology.org/nongmoshoppingguide
26. http://www.myersbriggs.org/
27. http://psychcorp.pearsonassessments.com/HAIWEB/Cultures/en-us/Productdetail.htm?Pid=PAg115
28. Http://www.mmpionline.com
29. Noakes, Manny; Foster, Paul R.; Keogh, Jennifer B.; James, Anthony P.; Mamo, John C.; Clifton, Peter M. Comparison of isocaloric very low carbohydrate/high saturated fat and high carbohydrate/low saturated fat diets on body composition and cardiovascular risk. *Nutrition & Metabolism.* 2006, Vol. 3, p7-13.
30. Kris-Etherton, Penny M.; Zhao, Guixiang; Pelkman, Christine L.; Fishell, Valerie K.; Coval, Stacie M. Beneficial Effects of a Diet High in Monounsaturated Fatty Acids on Risk Factors for Cardiovascular Disease. *Nutrition in Clinical Care.* May/Jun2000, Vol. 3 Issue 3, p153-162.
31. http://www.uab.edu/news/latest/item/2182-high-fat-low-carb-diets-not-for-obese-people-at-risk-of-heart-attack
32. http://www.drfostersessentials.com/store/juicing.php
33. http://www.cancer.org/cancer/cancercauses/othercarcinogens/athome/recombinant-bovine-growth-hormone
34. http://www.pbs.org/wgbh/pages/frontline/shows/meat/safe/overview.html
35. Michaels, Jillian, 2007. *Making the Cut.* Three Rivers Press, New York.
36. Lodge, Dr. Henry, and Chris Crowley, 2004. *Younger Next Year,* Workman Press, USA. The logic behind exercise for human health.

37. Campbell, Dr. T. Colin & Thomas Campbell, 2006. *The China Study*. Benbella, Dallas, Texas. The most complete book on nutritional health to date.
38. McDougall, Dr. John, 1994. *The McDougall Program for Maximum Weight Loss*. Dutton, USA. The weight loss diet and many recipes.
39. Esselstyn, Dr. Caldwell B., 2007. *Prevent and Reverse Heart Disease*. Penguin Group, NY. Nutritional methods for better health.
40. Ornish, Dr. Dean, 1996. *Dr. Dean Ornish's Program for Reversing Heart Disease*. Random House, USA. Nutritional methods for better health.
41. http://www.mfablog.org/2012/12/plant-based-foods-predicted-to-take-center-stage-in-2013.html
42. http://www.nydailynews.com/life-style/health/worst-fast-food-meals-kids-weigh-close-1-000-fat-laden-calories-study-article-1.453152
43. http://www.infoplease.com/ipa/A0934642.html

About Your Authors

Prianka Mansur is a nationally certified fitness instructor specializing in Pilates, and general health and well-being. She has spent most of her life searching for ways to better her body and life. After years of following a strict vegetarian diet, she found the numerous benefits of juicing. After months of research and personal experience, she has become an avid supporter of juicing, juice fasts, and a life incorporating a juice diet. She now lives along the Gulf Coast where she teaches belly dance and Pilates, enjoys jogging outdoors, and juicing locally bought fruits and vegetables.

Dr. Jacqueline Zaleski Mackenzie, has been eating naturally for health since high school when she lost an aunt to cancer. She knew her grandmother had died in her 30s of cancer. Both her parents died of cancer. At age 19, "Jacquie" gave birth to an infant, who had congenital defects. Using totally natural foods and a non-chemical based medicine that simply slowed her heart rate (digitalis) so the heart muscle could heal; by the age of 4 the defect was gone. The medical community called it "a miracle."

Jacquie has grown her own organic foods since 1969, has fasted since 1976, left a meat diet in

1979, and takes no medication: food is her medicine. She offers equine therapy and water therapy to marginalized children in an indigenous village as her doctorate is in special education, bilingual education and socio-cultural studies. She teaches local people through example that the vegan lifestyle and organic raw food are an inexpensive alternative to toxic medications. Finally, dances the Zumba with the indigenous grade-school students who she serves as a volunteer English teacher in Central Mexico. Her weight and overall fitness are better at age 66 than at her age 15. Her passion is writing about natural health and fitness options "on a budget" for any age.

www.ingramcontent.com/pod-product-compliance
Lightning Source LLC
Chambersburg PA
CBHW050421290526
45786CB00003B/1354